First published 2008
© Cyril Francis, 2008

COUNTRYSIDE BOOKS
3 Catherine Road
Newbury, Berkshire

To view our complete range of books,
please visit us at
www.countrysidebooks.co.uk

ISBN 978 1 84674 085 5

*Cover picture of Walberswick
supplied by Robert Hallmann*

Photographs by the author
Maps by CJWT Solutions

Designed by Peter Davies, Nautilus Design

Produced through MRM Associates Ltd, Reading
Typeset by CJWT Solutions, St Helens
Printed in Thailand

Contents

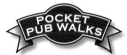

POCKET
PUB WALKS

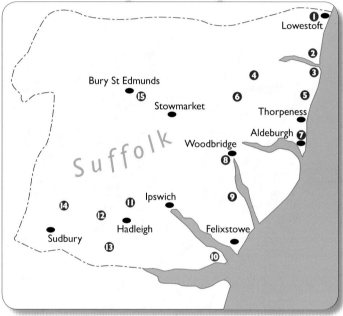

Lowestoft

❶
❷
❸

Bury St Edmunds

❹

⓯

Stowmarket

❻

❺

Thorpeness

Aldeburgh ❼
❼

Woodbridge

Suffolk

❽

❾

⑪ Ipswich

⓮

⑫

Felixstowe

Sudbury

Hadleigh

⑬

⑩

Area map showing location of the walks

Introduction

Suffolk is a great place to combine a relaxing walk with a visit to a welcoming pub The hostelries featured in this book come in all shapes, sizes and age. Some are located in idyllic surroundings by a riverside, on a village green, along the coast or in a town area. They all have one thing at least in common – they provide sustenance and relaxation for hungry walkers. What better after a walk than to reward yourself with a hearty meal or a thirst-quenching beer?

Talking of beer and the smell of hops, did you know that Suffolk has two of the oldest and biggest breweries in the land, namely Greene King (established in 1799) and Adnams (established in 1872)? Some pubs recommended in the book carry Greene King's IPA and Old Speckled Hen, along with Adnams Best Bitter and Broadside, plus a selection of other real ales and beers.

Walk routes in Suffolk may lack the drama of mountain-top vistas or rugged moorland but any shortfall is more than made up by the rich variety of wildlife, history and landscape. Few other places can rival the county in terms of a coastline designated as being of outstanding natural beauty, a quintessential seaside resort like Southwold, historic towns such as Aldeburgh and Woodbridge, quiet riverside harbours, grand churches and picturesque villages – all of which are featured in the book.

Although most of the walking is along the flat, there are some gentle slopes and the occasional sharp incline, but nothing too strenuous. You may consider taking appropriate clothing and footwear on the walk since there is precious little shelter in some places and paths often become muddy. A copy of the relevant Ordnance Survey map is always handy to carry, especially if you require greater clarification of the route or want to join up with other walks in the local area.

Although the information contained in the book is believed to be up to date, it's best to contact individual landlords in advance regarding pub opening times, food and parking. Most will let you use the pub yard if requested and it goes without saying that you should also be a customer.

Cyril Francis

Publisher's Note

We hope that you obtain considerable enjoyment from this book; great care has been taken in its preparation. However, changes of landlord and actual closures are sadly not uncommon. Likewise, although at the time of publication all routes followed public rights of way or permitted paths, diversion orders can be made and permissions withdrawn.

We cannot, of course, be held responsible for such diversion orders and any inaccuracies in the text which result from these or any other changes to the routes nor any damage which might result from walkers trespassing on private property. We are anxious though that all details covering the walks are kept up to date and would therefore welcome information from readers which would be relevant to future editions.

The simple sketch maps that accompany the walks in this book are based on notes made by the author whilst checking out the routes on the ground. However, for the benefit of a proper map, we do recommend that you purchase the relevant Ordnance Survey sheet covering your walk. The Ordnance Survey maps are widely available, especially through booksellers and local newsagents.

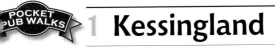

1 Kessingland

The King's Head

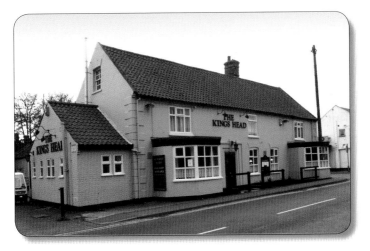

Coast and countryside just about sums up this entertaining route. The walk is on the so-called touristy sunrise coast. Walk here during the season, particularly at weekends, and you'll often find parts of Kessingland crowded with holidaymakers. However, walk during off-peak periods and you have the broad area of sand dunes almost to yourself. On a clear day there are grand views of the North Sea coastline, especially north towards the cliffs at Pakefield and the holiday resort of Lowestoft.

Elsewhere there is some delightful countryside walking, where the 98 ft tower of St Edmund's church acts as a useful landmark.

Suffolk

Distance – 3 miles.

OS Explorer 231 Southwold & Bungay GR 524866.
There are no stiles on the walk, which chiefly follows tracks,
field paths and a stretch of coastline.

Starting point The King's Head, 66 High Street, Kessingland.

How to get there Kessingland is some 5 miles south
of Lowestoft. From Lowestoft take the A12 and leave at
roundabouts located at either end of the Kessingland by-pass.
Follow signs to the High Street as directed. Park in the pub car
park with the landlord's permission.

From details contained on information panels passed during the
walk, you learn that Sir Henry Rider Haggard, author of such
celebrated books such as *King Solomon's Mines* and *She*, once had
a house on the cliffs. Strangely enough, when it came to fishing,
Kessingland was more important than Lowestoft. At one time
the village paid a rent of 22,000 live herrings to the Crown.

THE PUB The **King's Head** stands beside what was once the A12
main road to Lowestoft. You can take meals in the spacious
bar area or in the restaurant. Traditional pub grub on offer
includes dishes such as lasagne, chilli, scampi, curries, steaks
and burgers. Sandwiches and children's portions are available.
On Tuesday and Thursday there are specials for senior citizens,
well worth the money. A large selection of beers and ales includes
Guinness, John Smiths, Tetley, Carlsberg and Kronenbourg, plus
a range of wines.

*The pub is open all week from 11 am to 11 pm. Food is served
daily, except Mondays and Wednesdays from 12 noon to 3 pm
and 6.30 pm to 9 pm.* ☎ 01502 740252

Kessingland (Walk 1)

1 Leave the pub car park and walk north-east along the High Street. Pass Field Lane where the High Street becomes the London Road. Continue past the houses on the right and when you reach house **No 109** on the left, turn right through a hedge gap to join a well-worn permissive field edge path.

2 Stay on the path as it winds its way forward to meet a path coming from the left - the **Suffolk Coast and Heaths Path**. Follow the latter up to and then through the woods ahead to meet a stony track. Turn right and continue parallel to the cliff top. There are one or two opportunities to turn left to the beach area if desired.

3 The track now becomes surfaced at odd intervals. Where the road turns right, continue straight ahead along **Green Lane** and another stony surface. Pass the site of Kessingland cottages and holiday chalets and in about another 250 yards turn left into **Coastguard Lane**. Follow the narrow path to the boundary and

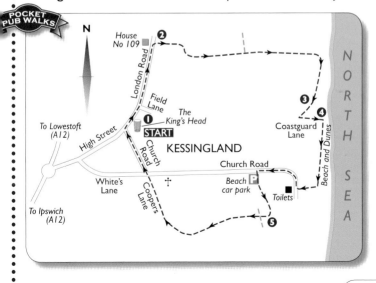

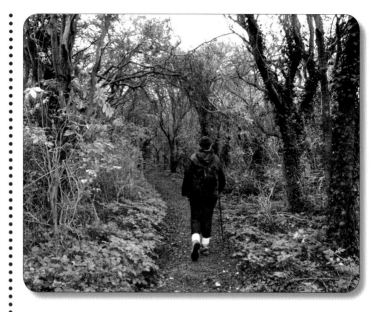

The woodland walk near Kessingland.

go down a flight of steep steps with metal handrails to reach the extensive sand dunes and beach. There is usually a smattering of fishermen present, trying their luck for catches in the North Sea.

4 Turn right and continue on a broad concreted path. Swing right at the far end to join Church Road with some public toilets on the left. Stay on the road for another 300 yards and turn left into the beach car park. Cross to the far side, go down a grassy bank and turn left. Pass between houses and a field along a green corridor known as Marsh Lane. Follow a broad access track ahead past a sewage pumping station and shortly reach a gate marked 'Private-Keep Out,' with a fishing lake beyond. Keep forward for another 50 yards, turn right through a gap in the hedge and walk up the right edge of a cultivated field.

5 Pass over a track called **New Road** and continue ahead on a grassy path with hedgerows either side. Follow the waymarker posts as the path becomes narrower and a field edge appears on the right. Pass a fingerpost and carry on straight ahead. A water tower soon appears in the top left corner and the track, known as **Cooper's Lane**, now becomes surfaced. Carry on up the rising lane to reach the junction with **Church Road** and **White's Lane**. Cross the road and swing left and right into **Church Road**. Follow the latter to the **High Street** ahead and turn right beside the **King's Head**.

Places of interest nearby

The **Lowestoft and East Suffolk Maritime Museum** in Whapload Road, Lowestoft, has a rich collection of ship models, fishing and ship artefacts, paintings and photographs. A traditional museum with something of interest for all ages.

☎ *01502 561963*

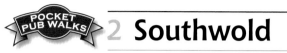

2 **Southwold**

The Harbour Inn

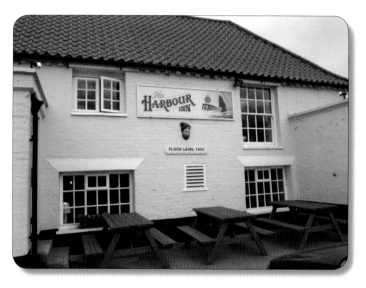

This absorbing walk gives a view of the seaside town of Southwold. The circular route takes you over the marshes to the rear of the town, past the pier, along the promenade or cliff, through the sand dunes and back to the riverside. Along the way you pass some of the famous beach huts, with amusing names such as Goosebumps, The Great Escape, Kippers In A Box and Albert Road, etc. Unlike some of its coastal neighbours, Southwold has managed to retain an old-fashioned genteel nature, unspoilt and refusing to succumb to modernity. No fast

Distance – 4 miles.

OS Explorer 231 Southwold & Bungay GR 501750.
A mixture of marshland paths and sandy dunes with stretches of surfaced roads.

Starting point Outside the Harbour Inn at Blackshore, Southwold.

How to get there Coming from Ipswich on the A12, turn right just north of Blythburgh to join the A1095. Follow the latter over Might's Bridge and in another 500 yards turn right beside the King's Head pub to join York Road. Follow the latter down the hill to reach the Harbour Inn at Blackshore just around the corner opposite the river. Park on the Blackshore, opposite the river.

food outlets or kiss-me-quick hats here. It's little wonder that Southwold was once voted the UK's most quintessential holiday resort. When asked why they visit Southwold, most people mention the fine beaches, the little pubs and the local Adnams Brew, open green spaces, the pier – 623 ft of wacky amusements – and of course the countryside walks.

THE PUB One of the first things you notice on approaching the **Harbour Inn** is a mark on the wall showing the high tide mark reached during the disastrous east coast floods of 1953. Similarly in November 2006 the pub's kitchens and bars were flooded by a high tide. The lowest bar had floodwaters waist high but the pub has now fully recovered. In the popular restaurant you have the choice of dishes such as traditional fish and chips, lasagne with garlic bread, scampi and cottage pie. There is alternative seating in a large extension overlooking the river with views across the marshes. Drinks include the usual Adnams favourites and a selection of wines.

Suffolk

Open from Monday to Saturday 11 am to 11 pm and Sunday 11.30 am to 10.30 pm. Food is served daily from 12 noon to 3 pm and 6.30 pm to 9.30 pm (Sunday 9 pm).
☎ *01502 722381*

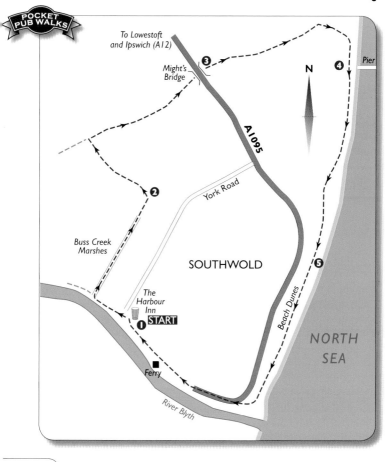

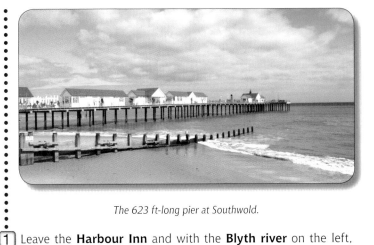

The 623 ft-long pier at Southwold.

[1] Leave the **Harbour Inn** and with the **Blyth river** on the left, continue ahead to draw level with the **Bailey Bridge** and arrive at a footpath junction. The intended way forward is over a stile in front and then over **Buss Creek marshes**. However, at the time of walking, this path was closed due to path erosion. An alternative option is to turn right and continue walking up a narrow, partially-surfaced lane. In front of you are views of Southwold's lighthouse, a water tower and the 100 ft flint tower of St Edmund's church.

[2] When you reach a four-fingered signpost, there is a choice of two routes depending on whether or not the way before you is flooded. *For the regular route*, take the left turn signposted to St Felix. Continue along the path and shortly turn right to join what was to be the original choice of path. Stay on this path that passes through an area of rushes and reed beds to give a rear view of Southwold. Horses and cattle can often be seen grazing on the marshes. Keep forward for another 800 yards or so to meet **Might's Bridge** at right angles. *If you wish to take the alternative route*, continue between gorse-laden embankments and later pass between a gap in a rail fence. Turn right and

Suffolk

follow a path through a stretch of gorse and afterwards continue along the left edge of Southwold Common. Leave the common at Blyth Road, turn left and, after 300 yards, rejoin the main route at Might's Bridge.

3 Cross over the bridge and the A1095 – the only main road into Southwold - and maintain direction through more marshland along an embankment path, with views of colourful beach huts in the distance. Pass the boating lake ahead and emerge at the pier car park. Turn right through the latter to reach the pier.

4 Continue on the cliff-top path past places of interest such as the lighthouse, the Sailors' Reading Room, South Green, and down the dip to the promenade. Go up **Gun Hill** and pass the six cannon looking out to sea, a reminder of the town's military history.

5 Maintain direction through the sand dunes or by the water's edge to finally reach the lifeboat museum. Turn right onto a road by the RNLI station and then swing left and right behind railings adjacent to the river. Continue walking along the firm stony surface, passing black-tarred sheds selling fresh fish and things nautical back to your starting point just ahead on the right.

Place of interest nearby

In **Southwold** itself there are several attractions including the Amber Shop and Museum, the Sailors' Reading Room, Lifeboat Museum and pier. Inland further down the coast is **Snape Maltings**, a unique collection of Victorian buildings nestling beside the river Alde, where barley was once malted for the brewing trade. Nowadays the site is filled with shops and galleries, with the well-known Snape Concert Hall located nearby.
☎ 01728 688303

3 Walberswick

The Anchor Inn

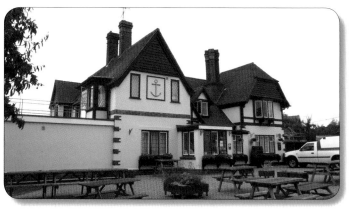

This relatively short walk takes you through and around the attractive village of Walberswick. You can catch the ferry (a small rowing boat) to cross the tidal river Blyth and do the Southwold walk as well, or vice versa. The ferry came into existence in 1236 and has been run by the same family for over 70 years. You can also catch crabs at Walberswick. The British Crabbing Championships are held here annually in August when children compete to catch the largest specimen.

The picturesque area, with its harbour, river and coastal surroundings, has drawn artists from a wide area over the last two centuries. Among the best known is Philip Wilson Steer (1860-1942), described as one of the few English impressionist painters. Prints of Steer's paintings such as *The Beach at Walberswick, Beach*

Suffolk

Distance – 2 miles.

OS Explorer 231 Southwold & Bungay GR 498745.
No field edge paths on this route, mainly good underfoot.

Starting point The Anchor Inn or Ferry Road car park.

How to get there *From the Ipswich and Lowestoft directions turn off the A12 south of Blythburgh and join the B1387 signposted to Walberswick. Follow the road through the village and find the Anchor pub at the far end on the right. Park in the pub car park with the landlord's permission. The yard gets quite busy during the season and you may consider parking in one of public car parks (fee payable) in Ferry Road, just beyond the village common.*

Huts at Walberswick and *Knucklebones* remain popular favourites and can be obtained locally. Nowadays the quaint village and surrounding area is under renewed threat of flooding due to tidal surges and defences being breached. In some instances, footpaths have been affected. Where possible, remedial action is being taking.

THE PUB The **Anchor** pub prides itself in sourcing local suppliers for its fresh seasonal food. Apparently some of the vegetables are grown and harvested from the pub's garden allotment. Dishes on the changing menu include the likes of Irish stew, fish and chips, fish pie, veal steaks and ham, bubble and squeak. There is also a vegetarian option. Desserts on offer include chocolate pudding, syrup sponge and apple tart. Adnams Bitter and Broadside are popular here and wine is available by the glass or bottle. Walk here during the end of November and beginning of December (check dates with pub) and you have the added bonus of attending a beer and old ale festival.

Open 11 am to 4 pm and 6 pm to 11 pm every day except
Sunday (10 pm). Food is served from 12 noon to 2.45 pm and
from 6.30 pm to 9 pm.
☎ 01502 722112

1 From the **Anchor** make your way along the road, passing the
public toilets and thatched shelter on the right. Continue past
the village sign and cross the common to reach some car park
areas either side of the road. The fishermen's huts and wooden
buildings of all sorts of designs and sizes that line the harbour
are present-day reminders of when the fishing and shipbuilding
industries were once a source of local wealth. The port, like

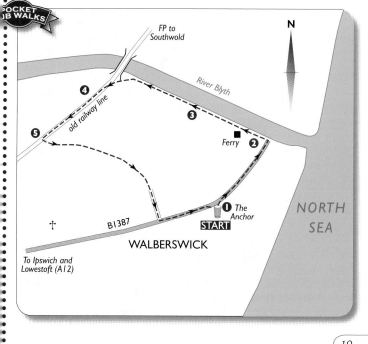

Suffolk

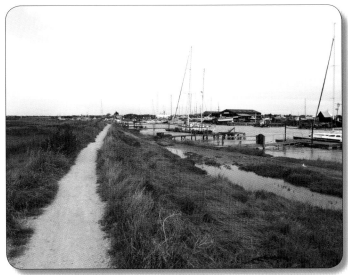

The path beside the river Blyth.

its commercial rival Southwold the other side of the river, has experienced fluctuating fortunes over the centuries due to a changing tideline and silted-up harbour.

2 Veer left towards the **river Blyth** to join the narrow **Suffolk Coast and Heaths Path** running beside the ferry hut. If you wish to catch a boat across the river to **Southwold**, the small jetty is situated almost opposite.

3 Continue ahead walking parallel to the river to pass a variety of fishing vessels, yachts and motor cruisers moored alongside the bank. At the boundary, you can also visit **Southwold** by turning right and crossing the bridge. However, for the purposes of this walk, turn left and continue on a metalled surface along the line of what was once the unique narrow-gauge **Southwold railway**.

The railway was built in 1879 with a 3 ft gauge and linked Southwold to Halesworth and the main line to Ipswich. Recently there have been attempts to revive the line but any hopes have been dashed due to opposition mainly from landowners and conservationists.

4 Later on, after passing between hedgerows of bramble and bracken, the distant tower of **St Andrew's church**, built within the ruins of an earlier church, appears – seemingly floating above the marshes. Look to the right-hand side for a bench beside the road. A metal plaque on the bench tells you that this is the site where Walberswick station – one of five on the Southwold railway – once stood.

5 Carry on ahead for about another 300 yards. Just before approaching some houses, turn left beside a bridleway fingerpost marked 'village green and ferry'. Go down a slope and then enjoy a leafy path with trees hanging overhead, providing a delightful shady interlude. Ignore paths going crossways and pass some stables on the left and private tennis courts on the right. When you reach **Leveretts Lane** ahead, turn right and walk towards the road junction in front. Turn left to join B1387, the same road on which you entered the village. Continue for another 200 yards to arrive back at the **Anchor** on the right or alternatively Ferry Road car park.

Places of interest nearby

Dunwich Heath (National Trust) is one of Suffolk's foremost conservation areas. There are superb views here of the coastline along with beach, woods, cliffs and magnificent flowering heather.
☎ *01728 648405*

POCKET PUB WALKS

4 **Huntingfield**

The Huntingfield Arms

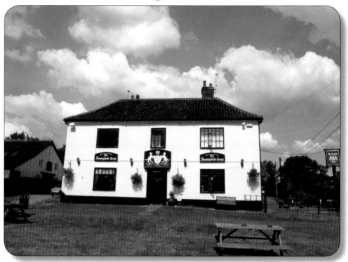

What connects a stately mansion, lush parkland, an ancient oak tree, impressive Huntingfield Hall and terrific home-made food at reasonable prices? The answer is a scenic circular walk starting from the Huntingfield Arms, set deep in the agricultural heartlands of high Suffolk. If it's country homes you're interested in, they don't come much more grand than Heveningham Hall. Work started on the hall early in the 18th century, with the Queen Anne centrepiece. Then, in the 1770s, owner Sir Gerald Vanneck commissioned designer Sir Robert Taylor to turn an ambitious vision into

Distance – 4½ miles.

OS Explorer 231 Southwold & Bungay GR 341738.
A walk through luscious parkland, but also considerable stretches of tarmac, albeit on quiet country roads.

Starting point The Huntingfield Arms on the village green. Park in the pub car park with permission from the landlord or beside the road.

How to get there *Follow the A1120 to the crossroads at Peasenhall. From here take the Roman Road to the B1117 junction. Turn right, continue on the B1117 (Halesworth Road) to reach Bridge Street on the left. The pub stands on the village green.*

reality. This involved almost tripling the length of the house. Capability Brown was hired to design the layout of the gardens and open parkland. Sadly the house is not generally open to the public and access through parkland passes only to rear of the house. Whether Queen Elizabeth I ever visited Huntingfield Hall and reputedly shot a deer from the shelter of a tree – hence the Queen's Oak – is open to question. True or not, the views here are some of the best on the walk.

THE PUB If you thought the **Huntingfield Arms** resembles a large house outside and in, you would be right. Some 150 years ago the estate manager of Heveningham Hall lived here. You can relax at a trestle table outside and gaze across the village green. Delicious home-made food features on a daily changing menu. Pies and casseroles are a speciality here. Other dishes include egg, ham and chips, lasagne and steak and kidney pudding. For drinks there are Adnams ales plus other guest ales and a good selection of wines.

Suffolk

Open Monday (not lunchtime) to Sunday from 12 noon to 11 pm. Food served is served between 12 noon and 2.30 pm and from 6 pm until 9.30 pm (no food Sunday evenings).
☎ *01986 798320*

[1] From the green in front of the **Huntingfield Arms** bear left and follow the road over a bridge and continue to the next corner. Turn left here and follow a track leading to **Huntingfield Hall** seen just ahead. Leave the track and turn right to join an ascending grassy path passing the hall on the left. Shortly the

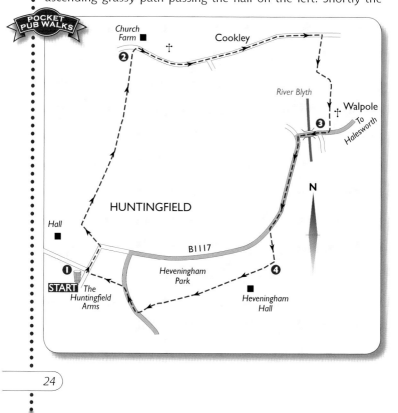

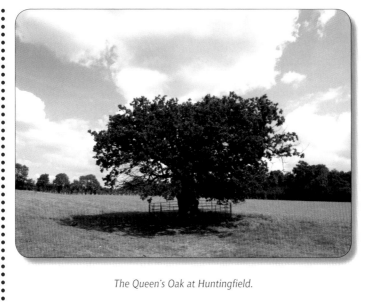

The Queen's Oak at Huntingfield.

Queen's Oak can be seen away to the right. The rising path soon passes hundreds of young trees planted in regular lines, woodland for future generations perhaps. Keep forward with a hedge on the left to shortly join a cemented farm road. Follow it to the road junction ahead near **Church Farm** and turn right to join a minor road.

2 Stay on quiet road for the next mile or so. Pass **St Michael's church** and later the **Cookley** village sign. Just after some houses on the left, look for footpath on the right. Go through a metal kissing gate to enter some rough pasture. Continue ahead and veer slightly left to cross a footbridge and afterwards a cart bridge. Turn right onto a narrow access lane just in front of a stable block and follow it to the road junction ahead to reach **Walpole** village. Turn right, pass the Old Post Office and ignore a road going left.

3. Continue ahead and cross a road bridge over the **river Blyth**. Follow the road as it curves left and stay on it for the next half mile or so. Look for an entrance gate and fingerpost in some metal railings and turn left to enter **Heveningham Park**. Follow the driveway down over a bridge with an ornamental lake appearing either side. Walk uphill and shortly turn right to cross parkland. Fine mature trees, plus young and especially tall weeping willows beside the path, provide a pleasant interlude.

4. Follow the fingerposts placed at frequent intervals to cross the park. Soon pass to the rear of **Heveningham House** itself. After the last fingerpost, aim for a gate in the railings beside the road and leave the park. Turn right and follow the road for about 120 yards and then turn left through an old iron gate. Veer slightly right and make for a stile. Cross the latter and proceed up a broad grassy stretch to cross a boundary stile. Bear right, continue along a stony track to find your point of departure a short distance away.

Places of interest nearby

The **Oasis Camel Centre** is a farm attraction with fun and interest for all the family. You can meet the likes of camels, llamas, alpacas, goats and donkeys. Llama treks can be pre-booked.
☎ 01986 785577

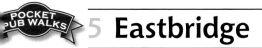
The Eel's Foot

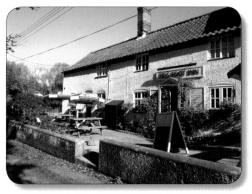

If you like combining birdwatching with walking, this is the walk for you. The varied route covers a habitat of coastal dunes, woodland and marshland. The Suffolk Heritage Coast has been designated as being one of outstanding natural beauty, unspoilt and little changed over the centuries. Starting from the Eel's Foot car park, a road and long track take you to Kenton Hills, where you continue along a popular route on permissive paths through Goose Hill woodlands, planted by the Forestry Commission in 1958. An area known as Sizewell Belts is a complex system of grazing marshes interspersed with ditches and narrow tree belts and is rich in wildlife. The walk continues through the dunes towards Minsmere, with the well-known RSPB reserve a short distance away. The return to Eastbridge takes you inland beside a drainage channel and over marshland, before you arrive back at the Eel's Foot.

Suffolk

Distance – 5 miles.

OS Explorer 212 Woodbridge & Saxmundham
GR 453661.
The walk follows broad tracks along permissive paths – not marked on the OS map – through woodland. Some paths may be muddy so stout footwear is advisable.

Starting point Th Eel's Foot car park. Park with the landlord's permission.

How to get there *From Ipswich take the A12 and leave it at Yoxford on the B1122 road to Theberton. In a further mile turn left and join a minor road to Eastbridge. Continue signposted to reach the Eel's Foot pub on the right.*

THE PUB The **Eel's Foot** is a pub where you feel you are taking a step back in history when you enter. The present building dates back to at least 1642 when it was originally two cottages. A third cottage, now the darts room, was added in about 1725. The pub's unusual name possibly derives from Eel's Boot, a type of woven reed basket used in eel fishing. Situated quite near the coast, the hostelry was once a haunt of both smugglers and parties of pursuing dragoons, who also needed rest and refreshment. Folk music is popular here with live sessions held on Thursday evenings. Delicious food served in ample portions includes beef lasagne, crispy whitebait, beef risotto, smoked salmon, barbecued ribs, and ham, egg and chips. A range of Adnams ales and beers is on offer, plus a varied selection of wines. Tea and coffee are also served. Meals may be taken outside or in the bar restaurant. B&B accommodation is available as well as a campsite 100 yards distant of Eastbridge Farm.

Eastbridge (Walk 5

Open Monday to Friday from 12 noon to 3 pm and 6 pm to 11 pm; Saturday 11 am to 11 pm; Sunday 12 noon to 10.30 pm. Food is available from 12 noon to 2.30 pm and from 7 pm to 9 pm, Thursday 12 noon to 2.30 pm and 6.30 pm to 8 pm.
☎ *01728 830154*

1 Come out of the parking area, turn left in front of the pub and continue up the surfaced road for about 400 yards. With a fairly new house away to the left (marked **The Round House** on the map), leave the road and turn left along a bridleway marked

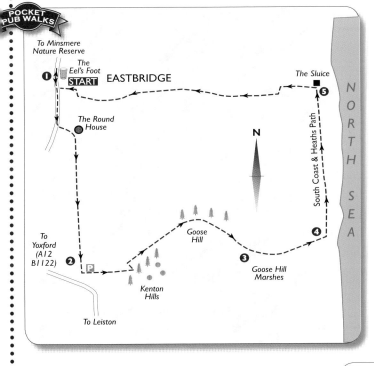

POCKET PUB WALKS

To Minsmere Nature Reserve

The Eel's Foot

START EASTBRIDGE

The Round House

To Yoxford (A12 B1122)

Kenton Hills

To Leiston

Goose Hill

Goose Hill Marshes

The Sluice

South Coast & Heaths Path

N

N O R T H   S E A

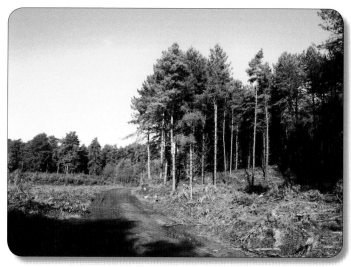

The track at Goose Hill.

with a silhouette of a nightjar, the symbol of the Sandlings Way Walk. Stay on the broad track for the next half-mile or so to reach the **Kenton Hills car park**.

[2] Go through a kissing gate in the north-east corner of the car park beside a covered notice board and take a descending path through the woods to reach a broad glade in front. Swing left then right to join a broad track running beside the left edge of the pine trees. A black band marks the route but waymark posts are few and far between. Stay on the track where it enters the woodland and shortly curves right with a high bank shortly appearing on the left, topped with a plantation of pine trees. Several trees have been felled here, leaving a large area of clearance.

[3] Continue ahead with **Goose Hill** grazing marshes appearing on the right. You may see ducks and geese feeding here. Shortly

veer right and cross a watercourse by means of a boardwalk, complete with handrails. Afterwards curve left beside a high bank on the right, maintain direction and finally reach the beach area.

4 You have a choice now of walking along the beach or through the low-lying dunes. Turn left and head northwards along the edge of the **Minsmere Nature Reserve**. Keep your binoculars handy to scan the marshes on the left as you walk towards Minsmere Sluice. Ahead in the far distance are the white painted coastguard cottages at **Dunwich Heath**.

5 Turn left over the brick-built structure that forms the sluice. Head away from the beach with a drainage ditch on the right. After about 300 yards the official path swings left and right, with the remains of a chapel seen on a hill to the left. Stay on the path and after about 400 yards, spot a large brick bridge away to the right. Just before reaching the hedge in front, turn left and right, then pass through a kissing gate. Follow the well-defined path that separates two fields and afterwards continue by a field edge. Where the path ends, turn left to reach the road. Turn right, continue along the road with the **Eel's Foot** appearing on the right.

Places of interest nearby

The **RSPB reserve** and visitor centre at Minsmere is just up the road from Eastbridge village. The reserve, which is open all year, contains a large area of reed beds, wetlands, heathland and woods. There are hides for viewing birds and wildlife, guided walks and a teashop.
☎ *01728 648281*

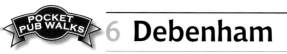
The Angel Inn

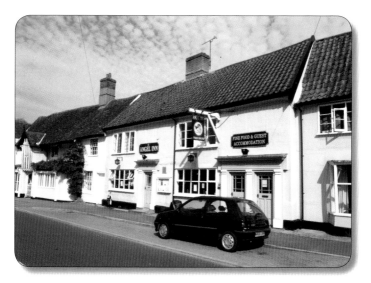

Be prepared for one or two ups and downs on this entertaining walk that takes you through the mid-Suffolk village of Debenham and beyond. There is a longer route and a shorter one, the latter ideal for family walking. After leaving the village, the route passes along the bottom of a deep valley, surrounded by large cultivated fields growing crops such as wheat and barley for local brewing. Hoppits Lake is an idyllic spot to pause and savour the local landscape. After visiting Blood Hall across the fields, there is a lovely broad grassy path on which

Distance – 1¼ or 3 miles.

OS Explorer 211 Bury St Edmunds & Stowmarket
GR 173634.
No stiles, mostly field paths and good tracks.

Starting point The Angel Inn at the northern end of
Debenham's main street. If there is a space available, park
in the pub yard (with permission). Otherwise park in a lay-
by at the front of the pub or nearby in the High Street.

How to get there Debenham is 11 miles north of Ipswich and
6 miles south of Eye. From the Norwich and Ipswich directions
take the A140 and turn off at the Mickfield crossroads. Follow
an unclassified road signposted to Debenham. The pub is about
halfway along the main street, the B1077, opposite Coleridge
Cottage.

to continue and afterwards a stretch of road walking. Debenham
takes its name from the river Deben, which flows through the
village via a ford, appropriately situated in Water Lane.

THE PUB Expect a friendly welcome at the **Angel Inn**, a 16th-century
inn and nowadays a restaurant. Traditional pub grub
is served here, including the likes of ham, egg and chips,
sausages and mash, lasagne and steak and kidney pie. Its
Little Angel dishes, containing smaller portions of main meals,
are a popular feature with families. Drinks-wise, the pub believes
in sourcing locally, hence apple cider obtained just up the road
from Aspall. Real ales include Adnams brewed in Southwold and
Woodforde's Wherry from just over the border in Norfolk. In
addition, draught Guinness, bottled beers and wine by the glass,
are also available. There is en suite B&B accommodation should
you choose to stay awhile.

Suffolk

Open 10 am to 11 pm every day except Sunday when it closes at 10.30 pm. Food is served from 12 noon until 2.30 pm and from 6.30 pm until 9.30 pm.
☎ *01728 860954*

[1] With the pub on the right, go north on the **High Street**. Just beyond **Old Toll House** over the road bridge, turn sharp right. Pass **Bridge House** and **Brook House** to emerge beside some metal railings with the aptly named **Water Lane** below. This is where the infant **river Deben** crosses the road and makes its

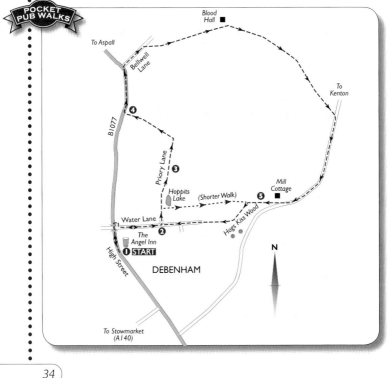

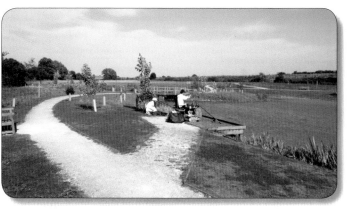

Beside Hoppits Lake.

way out of the village. Posts marked with depths of up to six feet give some idea of the water level after persistent rainfall and flooding.

2) Carry on for another 100 yards or so and turn left to join a surfaced lane posted as unsuitable for motor vehicles. Ahead is a delightful stretch of path with high overhanging trees. Pass the entrance to the village cemetery on the left and shortly arrive at the entrance to **Hoppits Wood** and lake. This is an attractive area created by the local community. With one or two benches positioned around the water's edge, this is an ideal spot for a picnic. *For the short walk,* continue to the top of the field and rejoin the route at point 5.

3) *For the longer route* maintain direction along the path which has now developed into an old earth lane. Shortly before it peters out, go left up some steps in a bank to enter a cultivated field. Bear right and take a gently rising cross-field path and head towards the boundary. With a ditch and uncultivated strip now on the right, keep forward and follow the field edge round to

reach a three-way fingerpost. Turn left here and with metal barns on the left, follow a downhill path that heads towards an oak tree and fingerpost at the bottom.

④ Turn right to join the **Aspall Road**. Continue along the road and shortly swing right onto a marked byway, **Bellwell Lane**. Take the next path going right, signposted to **Blood Hall**. Follow the gently rising access driveway, pass some farm buildings at the top and turn right as indicated. Shortly join a broad grassy path and follow it all the way to reach the **Kenton road**. Turn right and walk beside the road to eventually reach **Mill Cottage**. Just beyond the cottage, turn right onto a field edge path with a hedge on the right. The path eventually leads through a hedge gap to the field leading to **Hoppits Wood** and lake.

⑤ Here you have the option of continuing beside a hedge on the left that leads to a descending gravel track and some allotment gardens. A better choice perhaps would be to turn left over a sleeper bridge, pass through a kissing gate and enter **Hogs Kiss Wood**, an area of woodland owned by the Woodland Trust. Follow a grassy path through a plantation of young trees and leave it in the bottom right corner. Swing left then right and go right again at the next junction. Rejoin **Water Lane** and follow steps previously taken to arrive back in the **High Street**.

Places of interest nearby

Stonham Barns is a leisure, shopping and rural pursuits complex in the heart of Suffolk. It is located on the A1120 at Stonham between Stowmarket and Framlingham. There are attractions for all the family, including craft and specialist workshops, a golf driving range and flying demonstrations from the Suffolk Owl Sanctuary.
☎ 01449 711755

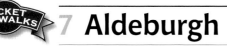

7 Aldeburgh

The Mill Inn

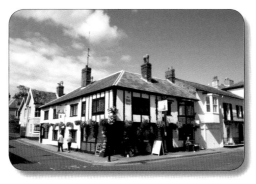

With an unspoilt coastline and bracing sea air, you can usually find keen walkers taking the coastal path, working up a healthy appetite in the process. Whatever the weather, this circular walk can be undertaken at most times of the year. Aldeburgh was once a small fishing village and later developed into a leading east-coast port. It was granted a charter of incorporation by King Edward VI and in 1571 it sent its first two representatives to Parliament, later to be disenfranchised by the Reform Act of 1832. Much of Aldeburgh's history can be found in a small museum located in the historic timber-framed Moot Hall. Built between 1520 and 1540 as a dual-purpose building, the ground floor was originally an open area for market stalls and the upper room has been used for centuries by the town council. It once stood in the town centre surrounded by narrow streets. Now, due to the encroaching North Sea, it stands perilously close to the shingle beach.

Suffolk

Distance – 3½ miles.

OS Explorer 212 Woodbridge & Saxmundham
GR 466568.
An easy walk out beside the beach and home along a dismantled railway line.

Starting point The seafront area in front of Mill Inn.

How to get there *From the A12 a few miles south of Saxmundham take the A1094 to Aldeburgh. Carry straight on at the first roundabout and proceed down Victoria Road. Turn left at the next road junction into Wentworth Road and then take the next turning right towards the sea front. The Mill Inn is situated just ahead behind the Moot Hall. Park in the seafront area or in one of the beach car parks.*

Further up the coast lies the fantasy village of Thorpeness. It dates from about 1912 and was designed as a fashionable holiday resort. A man-made shallow lake known as the Meare, has islands named after characters from *Peter Pan*. The village is a handy half way stop for light refreshments and toilets.

THE PUB The **Mill Inn** is a friendly family-run hostelry. Freshly-baked Cornish pasties are a speciality here – absolutely delicious. Along with fresh fish caught by local fishermen, other dishes on the comprehensive menu include roasts, steaks, ham, egg and chips and home-cooked steak and kidney pudding. The Mill also offers jacket potatoes and fresh sandwiches with a variety of fillings. Traditional ales include Adnams Bitter, Broadside and Explorer. The same brewer offers a good selection of wines. The small dining room contains paintings and photographs taken from local scenes. Booking is recommended during the summer season.

Open Monday to Thursday from 11 am to 3 pm and 6 pm to 12 midnight. Friday to Sunday 11 am to 11 pm. Food is available during opening hours but check details with pub.
☎ *01728 452563*

1 From the **Mill Inn** make your way to the sea front, noting the historic **Moot Hall** as you go. Turn left and head in the direction of **Thorpeness** along a tarmac path shared with cyclists. Fishermen, with their inshore trawling fleets, still work from the black-tarred sheds on the right; a scene made famous in George

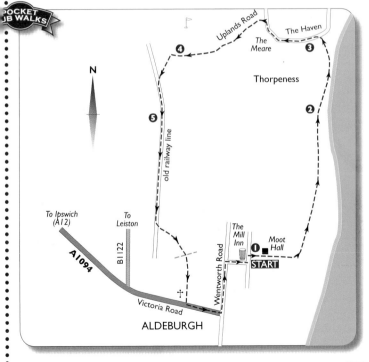

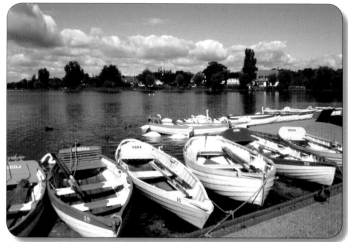

Pleasure boats beside the Meare at Thorpeness.

Crabbe's story of the local fisherman, Peter Grimes, best known as an opera of the same name by Benjamin Britten. Just ahead is a controversial sculpture in the form of a scallop erected in Britten's memory.

2 The surfaced path, that runs parallel to the stony beach and tideline, shortly peters out and is replaced with stony sections of heathland. Keep forward and navigate your way beside the beach to soon join some houses on the left. Continue for another 200 yards or so and look left for a raised boardwalk. Follow the latter, veer right through a car park and pass the village sign to enter the holiday village of **Thorpeness**.

3 On the left you'll find the Meare shop and tea room, with public toilets a short distance beyond. Keep passing the **Meare** on the left and soon walk beside a road called **The Haven**. Turn left ahead and continue along a track named **Uplands Road**. Pass

between a windmill (seasonal tourist office) and The House In The Clouds to reach a surfaced stretch of road at Thorpeness Golf Club.

4 Where the surface curves left, bear right downhill as waymarked. Keep forward along a path that continues beside the left edge of the golf course. Follow the path to a footpath junction, with **Meare House** (1882) appearing on the right. Turn left here to join the former trackbed of the Aldeburgh to Saxmundham railway line. The line opened in 1860 to transport increasing numbers of visitors to the popular resort. With traffic dwindling, the line finally closed in September 1966.

5 Maintain your direction along a permissive path, passing through the **North Warren RSPB nature reserve** as you go. From time to time there are opportunities for birdwatching between hedgerow breaks across the marshland. Pass through a gate and keep forward. Later on, the path enters a built-up area. Just before reaching a house in front, leave the main path and turn left to enter a caravan park area. When you reach a junction of footpaths, maintain direction to shortly pass beside the graveyard of **St Peter and St Paul's parish church**. Leave the graveyard by a gate; turn left into **Victoria Road** and walk down the hill to finally reach the **Mill Inn** at the bottom.

Places of interest nearby

Carry on further on up the coast to reach **Dunwich**. Located in a cottage in St James's Street is a small museum which is open from April to September each year. Inside you'll find a fascinating display chronicling Dunwich's disappearance into the sea over the centuries.
☎ *01728 648796*

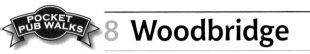

8 **Woodbridge**

The King's Head

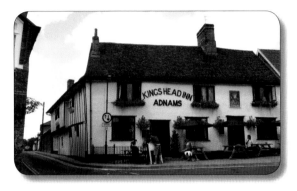

This compact walk takes you from the King's Head along winding lanes and streets through the thriving town of Woodbridge, where there are over 100 independent shops. From here, you walk down to the riverside and beside a picturesque stretch of tidal water to reach Kyson Hill which allows panoramic views over the town and river. The return to the pub passes places of historic interest, including Buttrams Mill, the tallest surviving brick tower mill in Suffolk.

During the 17th century, Woodbridge was renowned for its maritime trade. Local shipyards turned out sailing vessels for commercial owners and warships for the Admiralty. Nowadays, the town still retains its nautical identity, albeit on a much smaller scale. Boatyards by the riverside cater mostly for the leisure industry, including yacht and motor boat repairs, mooring and storage. By the water's edge, you'll also find an unusual white-

Distance – 4 miles.

OS Explorer 212 Woodbridge & Saxmundham
GR 272493.
Walk includes town streets, surfaced roads and tarmac paths.

Starting point The King's Head on Market Hill.

How to get there From the Ipswich and Lowestoft directions take the A12 which takes you along the Woodbridge bypass. At a roundabout on the outskirts of Woodbridge look for and join the B1079. Then proceed along the Grundisburgh and Burkitt roads to reach Market Hill in Woodbridge. Park in the King's Head car park with the landlord's permission. Failing that, there are parking spaces on the Market Hill (fee payable).

boarded tide mill. First recorded in 1170 and rebuilt in 1793, the mill is open to the public. There are ambitious plans afoot to allow the mill to work again and grind corn.

THE PUB The **King's Head**, which dates from the 16th century, is one of Woodbridge's oldest pubs. It looks out towards Market Hill and the nearby Shire Hall. You can take in the views by having a meal or drink sitting on the pub's veranda, complete with benches and parasols. To the rear is a small beer garden. Inside you'll find scrubbed tables with comfy seating, oak beams and a large crackling fireplace in the winter. The pub does sandwiches and light bites, plus a specials board positioned above the fireplace in the main bar. Favourites on the appetising menu include Cajun chicken, home-made steak burger, fresh cod and English sirloin and rib-eye steaks. There's a good selection of Adnams brews, plus seasonal ales and a comprehensive wine list from which to choose.

Suffolk

*Open Monday to Friday from 12 noon to 3 pm, 5 pm to 11 pm.
Saturday and Sunday 12 noon to 11 pm. Food is available from
12 noon until 2.30 pm and 6.30 pm until 9 pm.*
☎ 01394 387750

1 Leave the pub and walk down **Market Hill**, passing to the left
of Shire Hall. Continue down **New Street** (do not enter St John's
Street) to meet **The Thoroughfare**. Turn right, continue through
the shopping area and turn left into **Quay Street**, just past the

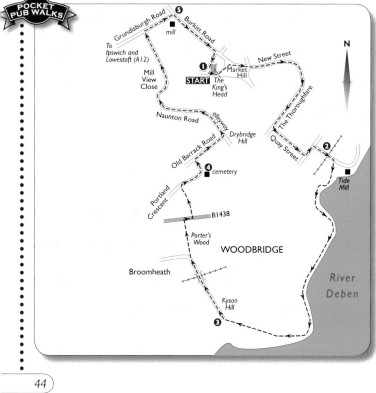

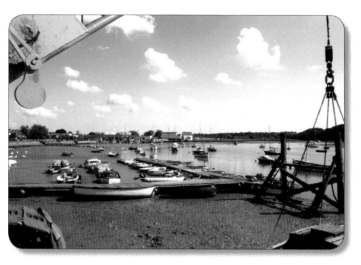

The scene along the river at Woodbridge.

Crown Inn. At the end of **Quay Street** turn left and after another 150 yards, cross the road to enter **Tide Mill Way**.

[2] Cross a railway line and make your way to the tide mill just ahead. Away across the tidal river and over the far bank, lies the great Saxon burial ship at Sutton Hoo. Retrace your steps and turn left onto a concreted path that passes moored houseboats and small shipyards. With **Woodbridge station** on the right, continue beside the river and make your way along the surfaced path. Hereabouts are lovely views of exposed tidal mud flats with moored sailing craft keeled over. Look out for swans and wading birds such as redshank and curlew. There are seats thoughtfully placed on a bank near the water's edge should you pause and admire the view. Keep following the path, later tarmac, to reach the National Trust's **Kyson Hill**. Go forward 20 yards up a slight incline and turn right to join a surfaced road.

③ Continue up the road, with its lofty views of town and river. Cross a railway bridge and afterwards pass a small car park at **Broomheath**. Leave the road where it later bends left and go straight ahead to join a narrow path beside a property called **Crosstrees**. A shady path now runs beside **Porter's Wood** on the right and terminates just before the next road junction. Turn right and continue on a footway beside the B1438. After about 50 yards cross the road towards some staggered barriers and continue up a flight of steps. A narrow path now continues between the back gardens of houses and emerges at **Portland Crescent**. Go straight down the latter and up the other side.

④ Turn left when you reach some cemetery gates and at the road junction ahead, turn right to join **Old Barrack Road**. Carry on to reach **Drybridge Hill**. At the bottom, with the impressive **Seckford almshouses** in front, turn left and pass through staggered barriers to continue along an alleyway to **Naunton Road**. Follow this to **Collett's Walk**, swing right and left beside **Mill View Close**, to reach the junction at **Grundisburgh Road** ahead.

⑤ Turn right and continue along **Burkitt Road**. On the right is **Buttrums Mill**, open to the public. Maintain direction and continue ahead to reach **Market Hill** and finish the walk.

Places of interest nearby

The National Trust's **Sutton Hoo**, which contains the burial grounds of Anglo-Saxon kings, has been described as 'page one of English history'. Explore the exhibition hall with a video and full-size reconstruction of a ship's burial chamber.
☎ 01394 389700

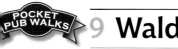

The Maybush Inn

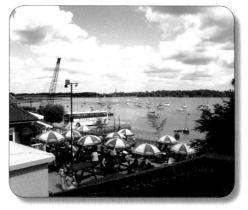

Your approach to the quay at Waldringfield ends suddenly at the bottom of a hill. Nowadays speed humps are in operation, otherwise the unknowing motorist might land up on the river foreshore or, worse, in the river itself. From the quay area, a narrow path meanders beside the Deben, taking in views of wildlife-rich mud banks and marshes. After leaving the water's edge, a leafy lane takes you back into Waldringfield village. The walk then proceeds mostly by field edge paths and stretches of road to Hemley village. Scenic countryside is to be enjoyed on this walk, with plenty of active sailing enthusiasts seen messing about on the river. Nearer the pub, there is the opportunity to relax on a short strip of sandy foreshore.

Suffolk

Distance – 2 or 5 miles.

OS Explorer 197 Ipswich, Felixstowe & Harwich
GR 285445.
A peaceful and pleasant walk along stretches of riverbank, open fields and leafy lanes.

Starting point The Maybush Inn.

How to get there *Waldringfield lies 8 miles east of Ipswich and 6 miles south of Woodbridge. Leave the A12 at the Brightwell roundabout and take a minor road signposted to Waldringfield. Follow the signs to the village and then proceed down Cliff Road to meet the Maybush at the bottom of a hill on the right. Park either in the pub yard (with the landlord's permission) or in the adjacent public car park.*

THE PUB

The **Maybush** is a pub with a view – and what a view! You can eat out on a multi-level patio and admire the peaceful scene across the river and beyond. What better place to enjoy a meal on a warm summer's evening? When the weather turns colder, you're welcome to sit snug inside by a roaring open fire. Food served includes dishes such as traditional fish and chips, seafood, fillet and rump steaks, a mixed grill, steak and kidney pudding and chicken curry plus vegetarian choices. Look on the blackboards for daily specials. Children are welcome here and have their own menu. Booking is recommended, especially at weekends.

Open: Monday to Saturday from 11 am to 11 pm. Sunday 12 noon to 10.30 pm. Food is available Monday to Friday from 12 noon to 2.30 pm and 6.30 pm to 9.30 pm, and all day on Saturday and Sunday.
☎ *01473 736215*

1 Walk down the entrance road to the car park, turn right and then left at the bottom. Continue for 75 yards, pass a boat yard and turn right as indicated to join a grassy path that takes you onto the riverbank (a flood-protection wall). Turn left alongside the river and follow it for the next half mile or so. Saltmarsh, muddy inlets and creeks accompany you as you make your way upstream

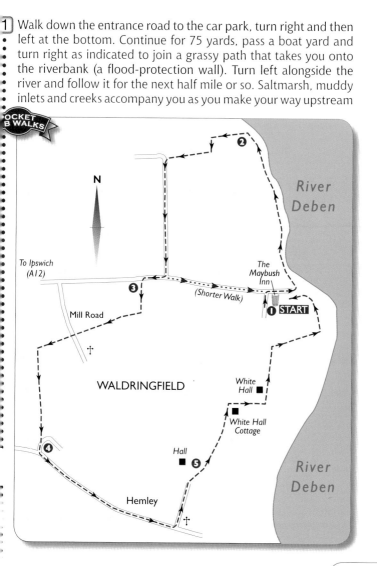

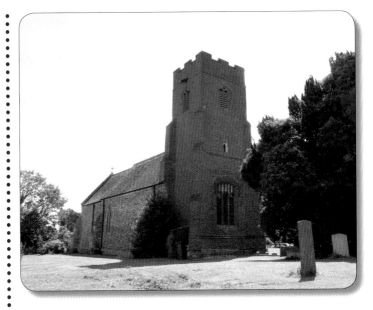

The church of All Saints, Hemley.

in the direction of **Woodbridge**, where the distant tower of **St Mary's church** appears in the top right-hand corner.

2 Turn left when you reach a three-way fingerpost and pass through an area of scrub. Shortly pass a dwelling on the right and afterwards join a track that leads to a public road at a sharp bend. Turn left here and continue along a quiet, leafy lane to reach the T-junction ahead. *For a short cut* turn left and continue down the hill back to the car park.

3 *For the longer walk* turn right and in about 20 yards turn left by a fingerpost and continue along a short stretch of access driveway. Swing right up a bank at the far end to enter an arable field. Take a cross-field path and afterwards continue over a green area

before passing through a hedge gap. Cross **Mill Road** and take the path opposite. The path initially runs between hedgerows and then continues beside a field hedge and then into a tree-belt. Turn left here, carry on through the trees and out into a field. Cross the latter, pass through a kissing gate and continue on a broad field margin to reach a minor road.

4 Carry straight on beside the road that soon curves left. In about 400 yards, at a junction, go straight ahead along the road signed to Hemley. Pass the driveway to **Hemley Hall** and eventually reach **Hemley village**. Immediately before the church turn left along a surfaced road. Shortly after passing a terrace of brick cottages, the road quickly peters out. Carry straight on here along a track with a hedge on the right.

5 Pass the house and farm buildings at **Hemley Hall** and veer right over a concreted section to resume the walk along a sunken farm track, lined at frequent intervals by pine trees. The track later develops into a stretch of concreted road that leads to a right-angle bend. Turn right, pass **White Hall Cottage** and continue down a leafy lane. At the bottom turn left, pass the boundary of **White Hall** and shortly cross successive arable fields. Swing right by a reservoir, pass through a hedge thicket to emerge beside moored sailing craft. Swing left and right in front of some chalet huts and out on to the riverbank and foreshore. Pass a sailing club building and afterwards go left up a flight of steps that finally brings you back to the car park.

Places of interest nearby

Newbourne Springs, just south of Waldringfield, managed by Suffolk Wildlife Trust, has a visitor centre and nature trails to explore.
☎ *01473 890089*

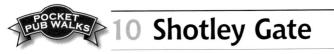
10 Shotley Gate

The Bristol Arms

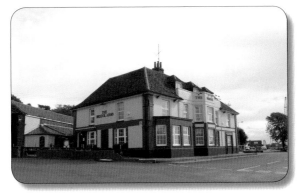

This action-packed walk on the Shotley peninsula offers plenty to see and absorb. Features include the confluence of two tidal rivers, an international ferry port at Harwich and the sight of some of the world's largest container ships entering and leaving the port of Felixstowe. The area has other strong naval connections. The HMS *Ganges* shorebase, which formerly stood beside the B1456 near Shotley Gate, trained generations of young seamen between 1905 and 1976. Memorabilia, including pictures and documents highlighting life at *Ganges*, is on display in the naval museum at Shotley Marina. From riverside paths there is the opportunity to watch small wading birds on the adjacent mud flats. Elsewhere, you'll find good tracks leading to higher ground where spectacular views may be found inland and over waterways across into Essex.

Distance – 3½ miles.

OS Explorer 197 Ipswich, Felixstowe & Harwich GR 246335.
Easy walking mostly on flat ground along riverside paths, with one or two gentle slopes.

Starting point The Bristol Arms at Shotley Gate on the waterside.

How to get there *Shotley Gate lies 10 miles south-east of Ipswich. Take the A137 to the southern end of Ipswich and turn at Bourne Bridge to join the B1456. Follow it direct to Shotley Street, and then to the end of the road at Shotley Gate beside the Bristol Arms. Park in one of the slots facing the river or alternatively at Shotley Marina.*

THE PUB The **Bristol Arms** is believed to date originally from the 12th century. It is thought that the pub was once the haunt of smugglers, especially with its direct coastal access to the Low Countries. From the bay-windowed frontage, it's possible to see the movements of ferries entering the port of Harwich on the far side of the Stour river. The pub is well known for its selection of sea food, including fish freshly caught further up the coast at Lowestoft. Other popular dishes include lasagne, toad-in-the-hole and a selection of home-made pies. Bar snacks and sandwiches are available. Drinks include Adnams Bitter and Broadside, plus a large selection of wines. There is a large patio garden where you can relax with a drink or meal.

Open every day from 11 am to 11 pm except Sunday 12 noon to 10.30 pm. Food available from 11 am until 2.30 pm and from 5.30 pm until 11 pm. ☎ *01473 787200*

Suffolk

[1] Start the walk by passing the pub on the left and continue along the road ahead that shortly bends left beside the water's edge. Away to the right across the water are scenic views of **Harwich harbour** and town. In front, the first view of the international container depot at **Felixstowe** comes into focus.

[2] Pass the entrance to the HMS *Ganges* museum and bear to the right edge as you approach **Shotley Marina**, surrounded by an array of boats, some placed on stilts for maintenance. Move to the front or rear of the marina reception building and Harwich Ferry departure point. Your arrival beside some lock gates may coincide with the interesting sight of yachts being lowered or raised between the basin and the river. Cross a metal bridge

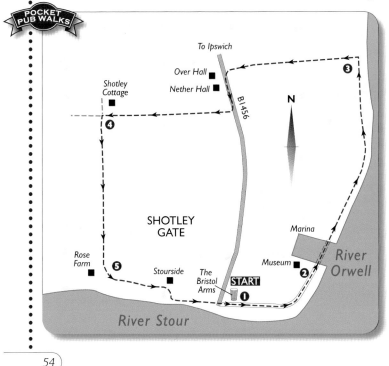

POCKET PUB WALKS

To Ipswich

Over Hall ■
Nether Hall ■

Shotley Cottage ■

3

B1456

N

4

SHOTLEY GATE

Marina

Rose Farm ■ **5**

Stourside ■

The Bristol Arms **START** **1**

Museum ■ **2**

River Orwell

River Stour

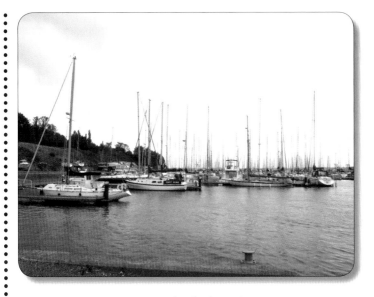

Boats moored at Shotley marina.

over the lock gates to access a broad path that takes you beside the **river Orwell**. Here, across the river, there are excellent views of ocean-going ships with stacks of container boxes being loaded and unloaded by large gantry cranes. The path soon bears left to meet a path coming from the left. Carry on ahead beside the river on a grassy path for about another 500 yards.

3 Look left, go down a bank as guided by a fingerpost to cross a bridge and stile. Continue over a stretch of marshland, where cattle may be grazing, to reach the far boundary. Cross another stile and head up a track and turn left at the top to continue on a footway beside the B1456. After about 200 yards, cross the road just before reaching a house on the right. Continue on a path to the right that runs beside a field edge and a hedge. Soon you will find the first uninterrupted views across the **river Stour**.

4 When you reach **Shotley Cottage** beside a junction of footpaths, turn left to join a descending track. As you make your way down, you'll find more superb views of the river, including roll-on roll-off ferries berthed at **Parkeston Quay** on the Essex side. At the bottom, turn left at **Rose Farm** cottages and make your way along a narrow path that runs between hedgerows and afterwards beside a field edge.

5 The path now climbs a slope to enter a brief stretch of woodland and emerges onto a road and houses at **Stourside**. Carry on ahead and then turn right almost opposite house number three. Go down a steepish bank and soon find a series of steps, which take you to the bottom. Turn left to join the **Suffolk Coast and Heaths** path. Across the mud flats at low tide you'll often find herons and small wading birds. Continue ahead and shortly pass a small picnic site to finally reach the **Bristol Arms**.

Places of interest nearby

Why not take the ferry for a 15-minute ride across the water to **Harwich**? Here you'll find a town and port steeped in maritime history. Attractions include two lighthouses – now turned into museums, a treadmill crane, the Ha'Penny Pier and the historic Electric Palace Cinema.

☎ *07919 911440 for ferry sailing times*
☎ *01255 506139 Tourist Information Office in Harwich*

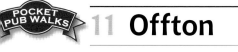

The Limeburners

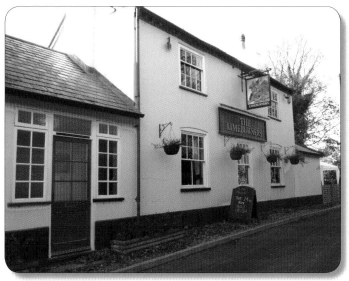

The pleasant countryside around Offton is uplifting in every sense. You may have to make a little effort on some sloping paths but nothing too strenuous. An idyllic stretch through an avenue of overhanging hedgerows takes you to the neighbouring village of Somersham. Offton village itself, contrary to popular belief, is not thought to have taken its name from King Offa of Offa's Dyke fame. Instead it seems likely that it was one of Offa's relatives or henchmen who had a castle (all but disappeared now) built on higher ground at the top of the valley, giving commanding views of the undulating landscape.

Distance – 2½ miles.

OS Explorer 196 Sudbury & Hadleigh GR 073493.
Mostly good paths, no stiles and generally well signposted.

Starting point The Limeburners in Offton.

How to get there *Offton is about 7 miles north-west of Ipswich. Take the B1067 and head through Bramford and then on a minor road to Offton village. From Needham Market, about 4½ miles, take the B1078 and turn off at Barking then follow the signposted directions to Offton. Park in the pub car park with the landlord's permission.*

THE PUB The **Limeburners** takes its name from a deep pit situated across the road. Chalk was extracted from the pit and burnt in kilns to produce lime that was used mainly for agricultural and building purposes. During the Second World War locally based US Forces used the pit for military training purposes. In 2006 the pub was temporarily closed due to subsidence from a burst water main. As a result, the Limeburners was refurbished with one or two new additions. The pub prides itself as being the only one in Suffolk with its own fish and chip shop attached. Other food choices include beef and onion pie, scampi, steak and kidney pie, chicken nuggets and burgers. Jacket potatoes come with a variety of fillings. For drinks there's a choice of real ales in the spacious bar area. You can enjoy your meal sitting either in the dining room, in the bar, on the veranda or in the garden.

Opening times: Friday to Saturday 12 noon to 11 pm. Sunday 12 noon to 10.30 pm. Monday to Thursday 4.30 pm to 11 pm. For the fish and chip shop opening times check with the pub.
☎ *01473 658318*

1. Come out of the pub car park, turn right and in 75 yards turn right again to enter an arable field. Continue along a field edge path that passes to the rear of the pub. When you reach a redundant telephone exchange building turn left, cross a bridge over a watercourse and turn left to enter uncultivated land. Follow a field edge path with a hedge on the left and later go through a hedge gap. When you reach a marker post bear right as indicated and follow a cross-field path that soon runs in a straight line towards the road in front.

2. Turn right on to the road and after a few paces turn left to enter the field opposite. Maintain direction and shortly ignore a path going right. Look left for some centuries-old Cedar of Lebanon trees, one in particular has a large girth with some of its branches sawn off. Swing right across a short stretch of arable field, pass under some power lines and turn left to join an old earth track. This, described on the map as **Chapel Lane Track**, shortly

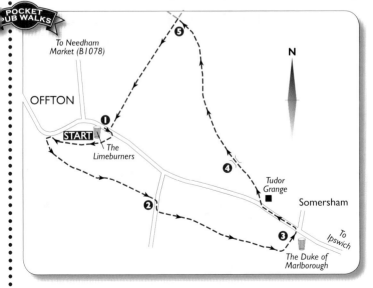

Suffolk

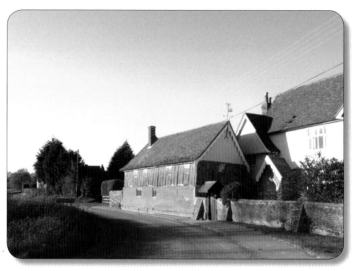

An old brick barn at Tudor Grange.

passes through a long shady area, with overhanging branches and a sloping bank on the right. This was once part of a highway network that linked neighbouring villages.

③ When you eventually reach **Chapel Lane**, **Somersham**, turn left and go past the chapel building to reach a road junction. On the right is another local pub, the **Duke of Marlborough**. Turn left, pass **Watering Close** and ignore a path going right just after crossing a road bridge. Immediately after passing a brick boundary wall at **Tudor Grange**, turn right and walk towards some farm buildings. Bear left as signposted and briefly follow a stony track. Where the track bears right, turn half-left and carry on straight ahead on a cross-field path that eventually leads to a wooden bridge. (Should the path not be visible on the ground, follow the earlier track for another 150 yards and turn left with the remnants of a hedge on the left.)

[4] Continue ahead on a short downhill section with trees and scrub now appearing on a sloping bank. Follow the curving hedgeline to reach the top boundary. Break right through a hedge gap, cross a sleeper bridge and turn left in the adjacent field. Continue with a hedge on the left, cross a further sleeper bridge and maintain direction down a descending path. At the bottom, look left for a bridge that takes you in to the next field.

[5] Continue down a gently descending path with a hedge on the right. Afterwards cross a grassy area and just before meeting a tiled barn, turn right to join a concreted driveway. Follow this to the road in front and turn right. The **Limeburners** is just ahead on the left.

Places of interest nearby

Discover facets of local history in one of Ipswich's entertaining museums. The **Ipswich Museum** contains a wealth of information about the fossils, rocks and minerals in the region plus galleries of British birds and Victorian natural history.
☎ *01473 433550*

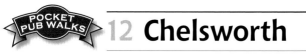

12 **Chelsworth**

The Peacock Inn

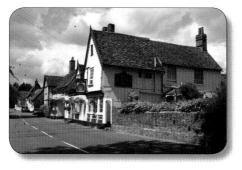

The quiet and attractive medieval village of Chelsworth lies quietly in the Brett valley. In 1959 it won the inaugural award for Suffolk's Best Kept Village. Little has since changed it seems. If anything, the village has got prettier over the years. Little wonder that artists can often be found here capturing the scenic beauty. The downside is a noticeable increase in the amount of traffic, being very much part of a local tourist trail, with Kersey and Lavenham not far away. Chelsworth is reckoned to have been the first ever village to open its gardens for charity. Some 40 years on and the village still opens its gardens to the public, traditionally on the last Sunday in June – a good time of year to visit Chelsworth and its surroundings.

The short walk takes you along almost the length of the village street. Field paths lead to the isolated church of St Mary Magdalene at Bildeston. Afterwards, a long descending path brings you back to Chelsworth and more glorious picture postcard

Distance – 2 miles.

OS Explorer 196 Sudbury, Hadleigh & Dedham Vale
GR 981481.

Starting point The Peacock Inn on The Street,
Chelsworth.

How to get there From Ipswich take the A1071 to Hadleigh.
Turn right on to the A1141 and thence to Bildeston. From
here take the B1115 to Chelsworth, about 2 miles. From the
Sudbury direction take the B1115 via the Waldingfields direct
to Chelsworth. Park beside the road almost opposite the pub,
with consideration for others.

views. Along the way there are houses, whose names such as The
Old Forge and The Old Manor House, denote a former usage.
Before starting or after finishing the walk, leave the car park and
take a short detour over the double-hump bridges on the left. In
an idyllic setting, water gently streams below a small waterfall,
with weeping willows lining the banks.

**THE
PUB** The timbered **Peacock Inn**, thought to have been named
after one-time village resident Mary Peacock, is conveniently
situated beside the B1115 in the heart of the village. Although
the pub might be considered upmarket with its main menu,
it does welcome walkers. Fresh sandwiches, baguettes and
ploughman's are available. The selection of light meals includes
dishes such as gammon steaks, scampi and chips, and steak and
mushroom pudding. There is also a good list of starters and
desserts from which to choose. Traditional roasts are available
on a Sunday. The bar offers an extensive list of wines, along with
guest ales and local beers such as Adnams, Greene King and
Woodfordes. Tea and coffee is also served. During the summer

months you can relax in the beer garden or sit by a cosy open fire when the weather turns colder.

Opening times: Monday closed. Tuesday to Saturday from 11 am to 3 pm and 6 pm to 11 pm. Sunday 12 noon to 4 pm. Food is served from 12.30 pm to 2.30 pm and from 6 pm to 9 pm.
☎ *01449 740758*

[1] Walk along the footway in the direction of neighbouring **Monks Eleigh**. If you wish to visit **All Saints church**, cross the road

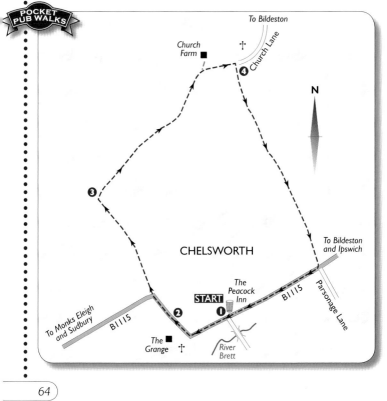

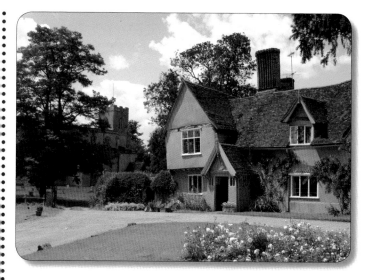

The Grange with church beyond at Chelsworth.

where it bends right and take the track past **The Grange**. The church is situated in a lowland setting beside a stream. You may find it locked but its unusual part-sandstone rendered exterior is worth a short detour.

2 Continue along the footway curving right. The village sign shortly appears on the left set back from the road. A nearby plaque gives a potted history of the village, listing its original name as Ceorleswyrthe. Leave the road where it now curves left and carry on straight ahead along a stony track.

3 After about 400 yards, just after passing a path coming from the left, turn right onto another field edge with a ditch on the right. Shortly cross a sleeper bridge over a ditch and maintain direction. At the next field boundary, turn right onto a cart track to meet a stretch of concrete at **Church Farm**. Turn right in front

Suffolk

of some farm silos and follow the path to the parish church at **Bildeston**. Just before reaching the boundary wall, note the path going right, your next path. Meanwhile, make a brief detour to view the church, which stands on high ground half a mile from the village centre. The church's unsought claim to fame is that its original tower spectacularly collapsed on Ascension Day 1975. Work on the modern replacement tower was finally completed in November 1999.

4 Return to the path noted in point 3 and pass through an area of part scrubland. Keep heading towards a hedge in front where you later pass through a gap to enter the adjoining field. Walk beside the field edge and carry straight on where the hedgeline ends. Stay on the lengthy cross-field path which gently descends to meet the B1115 opposite **Parsonage Lane**. Turn right to pass more period properties plus the **Victory Hall**, a First World War army hut, the village memorial of the Great War. Finally, keep forward to reach the **Peacock Inn** a little further on.

Places of interest nearby

Lavenham has a wealth of medieval buildings and a grand spacious church to explore. The early 16th-century timber framed Guildhall of Corpus Christi, later a jail and workhouse, contains exhibitions on local history and the cloth industry.
☎ 01787 247646

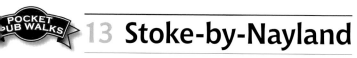

The Angel Inn

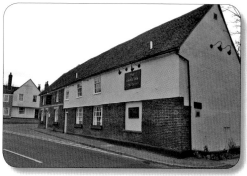

The tourist brochures often tell you that the impressive church of St Mary is not to be missed: excellent advice. Hard not to miss is the reddish brick 120 ft tower, standing on a hillside and seen for miles away. Stoke-by-Nayland, not to be confused with neighbouring Nayland, stands right on the border of Suffolk and Essex overlooking the Stour valley.

The route takes you by way of country lanes, field edge paths and pasture to the picturesque next door village of Polstead, often associated with Maria Marten and the Red Barn murder, a 19th-century melodrama. Climbing up the grass mound at Bell's Hill might need a bit extra huff and puff but is well worth the effort, if only to sit on a bench at the top and admire the glorious views across the Box valley.

THE PUB Expect to receive a warm welcome at the **Angel**, a traditional 16th-century coaching inn. Inside there are low

Suffolk

Distance – 5 miles.

OS Explorer 196 Sudbury, Hadleigh & Dedham Vale
GR 989363.
Some gentle slopes plus a steepish climb and descent at Bells Hill.

Starting point The Angel Inn at Stoke-by-Nayland.

How to get there *From the Ipswich and Colchester directions take the A12 and leave it at the signposted Higham turn off. Take the B1068 and follow it to Polstead Street at Stoke-by-Nayland, where the Angel is on the left-hand side. You can park at the pub with the landlord's permission. Alternatively, park in a side road or at the recreational ground in School Street.*

ceilings with exposed wooden beams, flagstone floors and partially exposed brick walls. During cold weather there is a roaring log fire in the bar area. The excellent main menu offers a choice of dishes such as beef Wellington, lamb shank, deep fried calamari, chicken liver pâté, haddock and goujons. There is also a specials board with other popular dishes. Drinks include a choice of Fosters, Guinness, Adnams, IPA and Strongbow, along with a good selection of wines. Tea and coffee is also served. B&B accommodation is available.

Open daily all week from 11 am to 11 pm. Food can be ordered from 12 noon to 2.30 pm and from 6.30 pm to 9.30 pm.
☎ *01206 263245*

1 Take the descending road signposted to **Scotland Street** and pass several pretty cottages as you go. After about 400 yards, turn left beside some white railings opposite a large thatched

cottage. Follow the narrow path across boggy ground, veering right to shortly meet a field entrance. Turn left into the field and continue along the left edge, soon going downhill.

2 At the bottom, turn left and maintain direction over pasture. When you eventually reach **Mill Road** ahead, climb over a stile and turn right. Continue ahead to pass over the **river Box** and in about 200 yards turn right. Later pass through a kissing gate to emerge into undulating pasture.

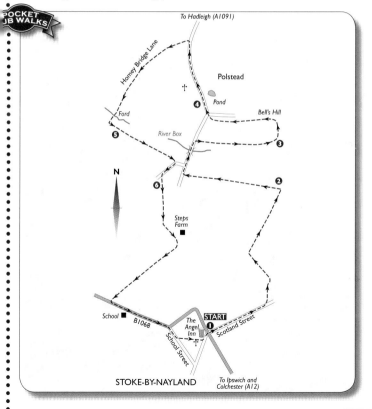

[3] Turn left and pass under some cables, then bear right and keep forward on rising ground beside a belt of trees. Bear left at a fingerpost and continue forward to reach a wooden bench. Descend the steepish earth mound at **Bell's Hill** and cross a stile at the bottom.

[4] Walk straight up the surfaced road, shortly passing a large pond. Maintain direction up a hill (to avoid oncoming traffic, you may consider walking along the right field edge as the locals appear to do). Turn left just before the road curves right to join **Homey Bridge Lane**. Continue down the earth lane, cross a ford at the bottom and turn left at a kissing gate.

[5] Continue along a field edge path, pass close to a weir and in another 200 yards break left through a hedge gap. Follow the path through a plantation and afterwards over rough grassland. Turn right at the lane ahead and in another 100 yards turn left up some steps opposite **The Thatch**.

[6] Continue along a field edge to reach **Steps Farm**. Turn right as waymarked across a strip of concrete into a field, swing left and left again over a short stretch of grass. Turn right with a hedge on the left and in 75 yards follow the path left out to a stony access track. Head up the track and later turn left onto the road. Pass a school and later turn right into **School Street**. Turn left again into a playing field, veer diagonally right over the field and look for a hedge gap into the churchyard. Leave beside the war memorial and head back towards the **Angel**.

Places of interest nearby

Bridge Cottage at Flatford (National Trust) contains an exhibition and memorabilia relating to the famous landscape artist John Constable. ☎ *01206 298260*

14 **Long Melford**

The George & Dragon

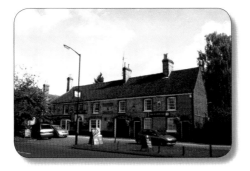

Long by name and long by nature might be one way of describing Long Melford. Despite having a 16th-century moated Tudor Hall, a grand church of cathedral proportions, a large green and a mile-long street all within its boundaries, surprisingly enough, Long Melford still officially retains village status. Either side of the main street, which you can explore at leisure, is a mixture of bakers, butchers, bookshops, antique shops and restaurants.

The walk initially follows a route that takes you to Liston Mill, just across the border into Essex. A delightful stretch then follows through water meadows beside the river Stour. The distant tower of Holy Trinity church can be seen on most of the walk, seemingly floating above the hedgerows. Later on, the route crosses the B1064 and proceeds along Bull Lane, where a path leads over an old railway line and eventually down an embankment and up the other side.

Distance – 1 or 3 miles.

OS Explorer 196 Sudbury, Hadleigh & Dedham Vale GR 862455.
An easy walk with few stiles, progressing along country lanes, water meadows and field edge paths.

Starting point The George & Dragon, Hall Street, Long Melford.

How to get there *From the Bury St Edmunds direction follow the A1092 and then the B1064. Carry on almost the entire length of Melford's main street (Hall Street) and locate the pub on the left. From Sudbury take the A134 or A131 and follow the B1064 past Rodbridge Corner. After another mile or so the pub is on the right. There is a car park at the rear of the pub.*

THE PUB

Standing beside the main thoroughfare through the village, the **George & Dragon** was once a coaching inn dating from the 16th century. Nowadays it is a popular hostelry for visitors and locals alike. Within its spacious interior, you'll find performances of live music on selected nights. Popular choices on a daily changing menu includes scampi, cottage pie, steaks and fish dishes. There are also daily specials along with a large choice of desserts. Beers include Greene King IPA and Old Speckled Hen. The pub also lists a wide range of medium to dry wines. Meals and drinks can be taken outside in a large garden and courtyard area. Bed & Breakfast accommodation is available.

Open from 7 am (8 am at weekends) to 11 pm. Breakfast is available from 7 am to 10.30 am. Food is also served from 12 noon to 3 pm and from 6 pm to 9 pm).
☎ *01787 371285*

Long Melford Walk 14

1. Leave the pub, cross over the road and turn left onto a footway. Pass **St Catherine's Road** and afterwards turn right to join **Liston Lane**. Follow the surfaced lane and carry straight on at the road junction ahead. Soon grazing meadows appear on either side. A raised platform, presumably used in times of flooding, is on the left. Cross the county border sign for a brief excursion into Essex and reach the weather-boarded **Liston Mill**, a former watermill.

2. Retrace your steps a few paces and turn left through a metal kissing gate to join the **Stour Valley Path**. Cross two bridges in quick succession over a weir. Continue beside the river's edge, cross a concrete plinth and turn right at the next marker post. Carry on ahead over pasture, keeping to the right of Melford's distant church tower and aiming towards the hedge in front.

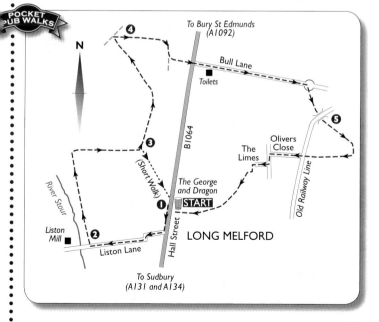

POCKET PUB WALKS

To Bury St Edmunds (A1092)

N

Bull Lane

Toilets

B1064

(Short Walk)

Olivers Close

The Limes

The George and Dragon

START

River Stour

Old Railway Line

Liston Mill

Liston Lane

Hall Street

LONG MELFORD

To Sudbury (A131 and A134)

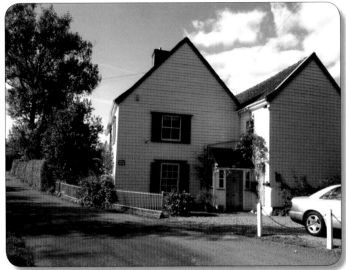

The old watermill at Liston.

Look for a depression in the ground and head towards an old metal kissing gate ahead.

3 Pass through the latter and shortly arrive at a point where the path divides. *If you want a short cut back to the start*, take the right fork, pass between the cricket and football pitches and afterwards bear left back to the pub. *Otherwise*, carry straight on to reach a staggered junction. Turn left here, cross a bridge and continue beside some garden allotments followed by a field edge. Bear right in front of a small area of scrubland. Shortly leave the path and turn right to continue along a bridleway.

4 Continue straight ahead and at the next footpath junction - the church tower now seen to grand effect on the left - turn right along an old earth lane where the hedgerows give a delightful tunnel effect. At the boundary, go left over a bridge and follow a brick boundary wall leading out onto the B1064. Cross over the road with care and continue along **Bull Lane** opposite. Stay on the footway, cross **Cordell Road**, with public toilets to the right. After crossing **Shaw Road** and **Lakforth Road**, continue almost to a mini roundabout and then turn right beside a RUPP sign. Follow a broad rising path through a housing estate to reach a bridge over the old railway line.

5 Continue to a field entrance, take a cross-field path and turn right at the boundary. Make towards the hedge, turn left and in a few paces turn right down some embankment steps. Carry on up the other side and pass to the left of a bungalow. Continue ahead onto a road (**Oliver's Close**) to reach a road junction. Turn left and quickly right and continue along a road named **The Limes**. At the far end, swing left and then quickly right into an alleyway. Follow the latter to emerge beside the **George & Dragon** to finish the walk.

Places of interest nearby

Gainsborough's House in Sudbury, birthplace of legendary artist Thomas Gainsborough, contains the largest collection of his paintings and drawings on display in the world.
☎ *01787 372958*

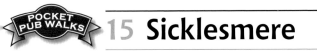

The Rushbrooke Arms

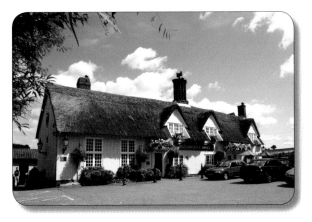

There are a number of interesting features to be found on this entertaining walk. For starters, there is a stretch of dismantled railway line. The single track, which was part of the Long Melford to Bury St Edmunds branch line, served several small villages for nigh on 100 years before finally closing in 1965. A small section of the former trackbed is preserved by the local council and passes through a lovely green corridor. Rushbrooke village was once an agricultural estate village and includes some attractive farm cottages. Nearby is a curious brick structure that apparently was once a well house. Visit St Nicholas church and you discover that, although the tower dates from the 14th century, much of the remaining structure is built of brick. Inside the church a Colonel Rushbrooke, who lived at the moated Hall

Distance – 4½ miles.

OS Explorer 211 Bury St Edmunds & Stowmarket GR 878606. Good paths, one stile and stretches of quiet roads.

Starting point The Rushbrooke Arms at Sicklesmere. The walk starts and finishes in the pub yard.

How to get there *From Bury St Edmunds take the A134 Sudbury road. After two miles the pub appears in Sicklesmere village beside the road on the left. Park at the pub, with landlord's permission.*

during the 19th century, undertook much of the alteration to the woodwork. The Hall, home of the Jermyn family for several generations, suffered a mysterious fire and was demolished in 1961 without permission.

THE PUB The **Rushbrooke Arms**, with its traditional thatched roof, dates back to at least the mid 18th century when it was known as the Wagon. Over the years the pub has been extended and refurbished. Part of a local granary barn was dismantled and re-erected and now forms a section of the restaurant. In the warmer weather parents can relax outside in the large beer garden with children enjoying themselves in an extensive play area. This family-orientated pub has a large choice of dishes on the menu. You can choose from the likes of steaks and grills, lamb shank, ale pie, lasagne, and sausage and mash. Look on the blackboards for the chef's specials of the day. Children's portions are also available. The bar contains a large selection of draught beers and ales including Carling, John Smiths, Kronenbourg and Strongbow cider. In addition, Greene King IPA and Old Speckled Hen are on offer. A comprehensive wine list is also available.

Suffolk

Opening times are Monday to Saturday 11 am to 11 pm, Sunday 11 am to 10.30 pm. Meals are served Monday to Thursday 11.30 am to 9 pm, Friday to Saturday 11.30 am to 10 pm, Sunday 12 noon to 9 pm.
☎ *01284 388242*

1 Facing the pub, turn right and walk up some steps beside a children's play area to enter a field. Follow the rising path under some cables to meet another path in front. Turn right and cross some rough grassland to shortly meet a thick rambling hedgerow

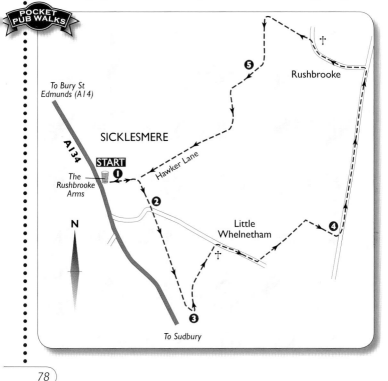

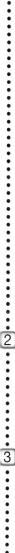

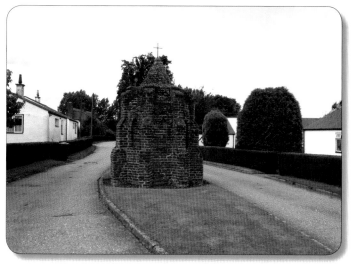

The curious brick well at Sicklesmere.

running downhill. At the bottom, maintain direction along a narrow path running between a hedge and a paddock fence.

[2] Cross the road ahead, go through a kissing gate opposite and continue along the former track bed of the Long Melford to Bury St Edmunds railway line. The path shortly straightens out and you are soon walking through an avenue of trees along an embankment with a bench thoughtfully provided should you wish to sit and pause awhile. Later on, the path goes up an incline and down the other side.

[3] Immediately before reaching a flat concrete culvert, turn left, go down a bank and cross a stile. Carry on with a hedge on the left along a rising path. At the top end, the path bears right accompanied by another hedgerow. Follow the grassy path to the far boundary and right corner. Go down a bank and turn

right on to the road leading to **Little Whelnetham**. Go past the church and shortly meet some houses on the left. Some 20 yards after passing a postbox, turn left at a byway sign. Follow the stony path, known as **Parsonage Lane**, between hedgerows and later pass a property named Nunn's Glebe. The path continues through a narrow tree belt and emerges at a road junction.

4 Turn left opposite a compound and continue along the straight road for the next 400 yards. About halfway down a hill turn left onto a road signposted to Rushbrooke. Follow the road past **St Nicholas's church** and later turn left to walk between some estate houses and a curious looking brick well. After passing the last house and a reservoir on the right, turn sharp left to join a cart track with a hedge appearing on the left. Keep beside a field edge and follow the track to an ash tree where the track almost peters out.

5 Keep forward for about 60 yards and turn right onto another track. Where the track bears right, continue straight ahead along a grassy strip. Look right and you may spot the distant cathedral at Bury St Edmunds with the spire of St John's church appearing almost alongside. Ahead are scenic views over the countryside. Shortly reach a lovely descending path named Hawker Lane, which runs between overhanging hedgerows, giving a delightful tunnel effect. At the bottom, enter the adjoining field and retrace earlier steps back to the pub.

Places of interest nearby

St Edmundsbury Cathedral. See Suffolk's cathedral in Bury St Edmunds, with its new Gothic-style lantern tower. Five years in the making, the Millennium Tower rises 150 ft over the central crossing of the building.
☎ *01284 748720*